*Stretch into shape*_____

by Tony Lycholat

Patrick Stephens
Wellingborough, Northamptonshire

First published in 1988

British Library Cataloguing in Publication Data

Lycholat, Tony
  Stretch into shape.
  1. Exercise 2. Stretch (Physiology)
  I. Title
  613.7'1   RA781

  ISBN 0-85260-006-3

Patrick Stephens is part of the Thorsons Publishing Group, Denington Estate, Wellingborough, Northamptonshire, NN8 2RQ, England

Printed in Great Britain by Woolnough Bookbinding Limited, Irthlingborough, Northamptonshire

10 9 8 7 6 5 4 3 2 1

Contents _____

Acknowledgements _____

In the writing of this book many thanks must go to: Monika Flooks for being a patient and willing model; to Pineapple Studios for the loan of clothing and footwear and to the editing and production team at Patrick Stephens Ltd.

Introduction _____

Up until recently, stretching exercises were not highly regarded in the fields of health, fitness or sport. Stretching was something that Yogis did, and was not for 'normal' men and women. Indeed, for a long time, stretching was accused of causing injury and making you 'too loose'. Yet as more and more has been found out about the human body and how it responds to exercise, regular stretching has come to be viewed as an integral part of all well-balanced health, exercise and training programmes.

This book is intended as a simple guide to stretching — a guide which outlines the real benefits of regular stretching. Methods of increasing range of movement and guidelines for postural exercises and pain relief exercises, all are discussed in the light of known anatomy and physiology: consequently, ground rules for safe, highly effective stretching are given along with programmes for various activities. Each exercise has carefully written instructions for correct positioning and maximum safe stretch effect. Everyone, whoever they are and whatever they do, can 'stretch into shape'!

Stretching — the benefits

Regular stretching exercises offer many positive benefits: a look at some of these will make you wonder how you ever managed without stretching before!

Posture and appearance

Although we often think of posture in terms of the upright body 'posture' can in fact refer to any position that we find ourselves in. For every movement that we make whether standing, sitting or in the field of sports performance, there is a more efficient way of carrying the body. This 'correct' positioning is what is meant by the 'right' posture. Not only does the right posture for any activity reduce the stress on muscles and joints, it also allows your body to work more efficiently and look better immediately, too. Postural exercises have often been called 'instant shapers' in fitness and health magazines, because they do just that. One major national magazine recently went so far as to say that sorting out your posture was the equivalent to losing ten pounds of fat in terms of appearance!

Most of us, because of our lifestyle, end up in one position for a long period of time — sitting at a desk, for example. It is common in this and similar situations, to end up in a posturally incorrect position. As a result of this, our bodies lapse into an habitually poor posture and changes begin to take place in our body structure: some muscles for instance, become abnormally lengthened, whilst others become abnormally shortened. This often means that other structures of the body can no longer work in the way they are supposed to. The poor posture we have adopted can in turn cause pressure on blood vessels, nerves, joints and ligaments leading to all kinds of posture related ailments from headaches to trapped nerves, sore joints and back pain — in fact, the list can be endless. Even the way you breathe and digest food can be affected if your posture means that the ribcage and abdomen are continually constricted by the way you sit, for example.

Appropriate stretching exercises can help you redress the balance and regain correct posture. The assessment section of this book will help you identify your weaknesses and then direct you to the right exercises for you. Where strengthening exercises may also be needed you will be directed to what is appropriate. Do also follow the guidelines for correct standing, sitting, etc, to make the most of your body!

Range of movement
Most of us take our current range of movement for granted and it is not until we are incapacitated in some way that we realize how important being able to move freely actually is — ask anyone who has any physical restriction to movements such as that which certain forms of arthritis bring about. Being supple or flexible means that you can reach, bend, twist and turn with relative ease. Effectively you can make full use of your body and its movement potential. Flexibility — which is what you achieve with regular stretching — is in fact a 'health-related' component of fitness (which simply means that an improvement in your range of movement can lead to an improvement in your general health and well-being). An increase in your flexibility makes everyday tasks easier to perform. Not only that but those same tasks also now require less energy to carry out than they did before you became more flexible.

Joint 'health'
Most joints in the body are designed to allow a certain normal range of movement, although this varies according to the nature of the joint and other limiting factors which are discussed in the next chapter. If a joint regularly goes through its normal range of movement, many of the joint's structures actually become stronger. This in turn makes the joint more functional and 'healthier'. Certain forms of arthritis can be alleviated through movement and stretching exercises, but check with your GP first, taking this book with you. Painful joints can also be the result of poor posture, so it may be worthwhile referring to this section of the book again.

Prevention of minor illnesses
Certain health problems can be posture related. Appropriate stretching will help relieve and prevent many of the problems listed earlier. Stretching exercises have also been used by many women with success to reduce and relieve period pains. Some people have also found relief from migraine and headaches through appropriate stretching.

Alleviation of stress
Stretching exercises can promote relaxation in many people, enabling them to cope with stressful situations at home or in the office.

Sports technique and performance
Just as posture can be more efficient, there is invariably a most efficient way of moving in sporting activities, referred to as being 'technically correct'. Many factors can affect an individual's ability to perform sports

related skills most effectively, but tight musculature inevitably limits range of movement. Many athletes owe their success, in part, to having an above average range of movement and more appreciate that increasing their flexibility means that they can apply force throughout the greatest possible range — as important to the sprinter and marathon runner as it is to the recreational competitor. Who does not marvel at Olympic hurdler and world-record 400 metre hurdler Ed Moses with his unbelievable stride length — or the fluidity of Sebastian Coe? Both are athletes who spend a lot of time increasing and maintaining their flexibility through stretching exercises.

Performing activities as correctly as possible reduces injury. Appropriate stretching can aid in the prevention of injury by allowing you to master sports or exercise techniques more fully.

Prevention of exercise injury
More articles have appeared in this country about the injuries associated with exercise than have appeared about the undoubted benefits of exercise, even though the reported incidence of exercise-induced injury is remarkably low. Having said that, injuries do occur in exercise, but in the main they are avoidable. One of the main factors in preventing exercise related injuries is a thorough and appropriate warm-up which incorporates some form of preparatory stretching routine prior to any exercise session. In effect, warming up prepares your body for an exercise session by increasing body temperature and taking your limbs, muscles and joints through their current normal ranges of movement. Such preparatory work has been shown time and time again to reduce subsequent injuries in exercise.

Prevention of muscle soreness
Everybody is familiar with muscle soreness and in particular that soreness which is associated with unaccustomed physical activity or exertion. Immediate soreness which occurs during the exercise or just after it, is due to an accumulation of by-products formed as a result of the work which the muscles have been doing. This type of soreness is best relieved by light rhythmical contractions of the affected muscles.

Muscle soreness which occurs at a much later stage, say at least one day after the exercise bout, is referred to as 'delayed onset muscle soreness' or DOMS. This type of soreness seems to be related to damage of the muscle or connective tissues. It can be relieved by warming the affected muscle, and then doing some light stretching exercises. Some authorities say and many practical examples have shown that to a large extent DOMS can be avoided and prevented if you engage in stretching exercises towards the end of your exercise session as part of a 'cool down' routine.

How to stretch _____

With all the positive benefits of regular
stretching exercises discussed in the previous
chapter, you probably can't wait to get started!
However, a word of caution: inappropriate stretching
is responsible for injury to muscles, tendons and joints.
There are certain guidelines which must be followed to get
the most out of any stretching exercise and to avoid injury.
The most important rules for safe stretching are the following:

1. All stretches should be anatomically possible

Stretching is easy. All you have to do is take a limb with its associated
muscles and joints to a position it has not been before. Yet all muscles
and joints have their limits. Certain movements are possible at certain joints,
others are not. Trying to stretch muscles and joints through ranges of
movement for which they were not designed results in injury.

The practical exercises in this book cover the major ranges of movement
at major joints. Of course there are many other exercises you could also
do, but for safety and effectiveness always follow the guidelines given here.

2. All stretches need to suit you

As with any exercise programme, the starting point is you. If you have not
stretched for a long time, or have not done any exercise of any form for
any length of time, do not expect to be able to do the splits!

The self assessment section on page 15 will help you assess your current
flexibility, and you should use this as a guide to your subsequent stretch
programme. Also bear in mind that flexibility tends to decrease with age,
so if you are older, do not expect to have the same degree of flexibility
as your children. Likewise, genetic differences can make some people far
more flexible than others. There are limits to everyone's range of movement
— be realistic. If your body will not allow any further increase in range
of movement, even though you are doing everything correctly, that's it.
Be content with where you are and exercise to maintain the range of
movement you have attained.

3. For the best stretch, warm up first

Warming up prior to any stretching or exercise programme is essential. Warming the body makes it more efficient in a number of ways: muscles can contract and relax more fully; nerve impulses can travel more quickly; muscles, joints and tendons are less likely to be damaged upon exercise; the response of the heart to exercise is improved; oxygen is made more available to the muscles for energy processes; warming up allows you to focus your mind on your subsequent exercise programme.

Many authorities firmly recommend that because of these and other favourable effects of warming up on the body, all stretches should be preceded by a general warm up period.

Warming up can be done in several ways. It is probably best to dress warmly in the first instance, by wearing layers of loose clothing — tracksuits on top of light cotton shirts are obviously ideal. Exercise in a warm, but well ventilated environment: the best type of exercise to do involves large muscles in rhythmical contractions. This means any activity like walking, jogging, stationary cycling, re-bounding, etc. You can do exercises which do not require any apparatus or lots of space and examples are given in the WARM UP section on page 17.

Using large muscles rhythmically increases the body temperature, as you will notice! You also need to include exercises which will take your limbs through their current ranges of movement as this prepares them for subsequent safe stretching. A good indicator of an appropriate warm-up is the onset of light sweating or glowing coupled with a general feeling of looseness of the limbs.

Most people can achieve these effects with about ten minutes of easy activity, although older or more unfit individuals may like to spend longer on this phase.

It is currently very popular to include what is known as 'preparatory stretching' towards the end of the warm up phase of an exercise class. All this means is that any muscles which are going to be used fairly strenuously in an exercise session are lightly and easily taken through their fullest range of movement. This seems to prevent injury. However, in an exercise class or exercise session, the bulk of the stretching work is best carried out towards the end of the exercise period, when the muscles are very warm indeed. There is no reason not to do both, though, including light preparatory stretching at the end of the warm-up phase, then the stronger stretches later on after the main exercise bout.

4. All stretches should feel comfortable

Whilst you will feel the stretch, you should never feel *pain*. Pain is invariably an indicator that something is wrong, or going wrong, in the body. if you have not exercised for a long time the stretches may be uncomfortable to begin with but they should never be painful.

If you do feel pain at any time, stop what you are doing and get specialist advice if the pain continues.

5. All stretches should be progressive

This means that you should always start with easier stretches first, then move on to more strenuous stretches later. Starting with a more intense stretch does not mean you will get results any quicker — in fact you may get the reverse effect since you may end up injuring yourself.

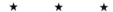

These are not the only rules. There are some equally important guidelines which relate to the speed of stretching exercises and how long each stretch should be held for. So heated has been the debate regarding these matters that the topic deserves a section of its own to resolve the argument: slow or fast, long or short?

Slow or fast, long or short?

Methods of stretching

How quickly should you perform an exercise and how long do you need to hold an exercise position for, are the most important questions in stretching.

At the turn of the century *ballistic* methods of increasing range of movement were very popular. As we have seen, stretching merely means that we have to take a limb into a position it has not been before. A ballistic method of stretching does this since you are required to force or fling out a limb to a new furthermost position. Such a technique of stretching is still very popular and works within reason. The major problem associated with ballistic stretching though is injury — to muscles, tendons and joints. This is because you are, in effect, asking your body to work against itself.

All muscles have specialized receptors built into them called muscle spindles. Their job is to pick up information about the length of muscles and how quickly they change length. They then feed this information to the spinal cord. If a muscle changes length very quickly, the spindle sends this information immediately to the spinal cord where a reflex response occurs. That reflex response is a command to a muscle which is being rapidly stretched to contract, or *shorten*. In other words, by trying forcefully and quickly to *stretch* a muscle, the body counteracts our wishes with a reflex action which *shortens* the muscle which is being stretched. The body does this to try and prevent major damage, but damage necessarily occurs the more force we apply. Sometimes we may only experience muscle soreness or tenderness as a result of forced or bounced movement, but real joint damage can occur as we cause the body to fight against itself. Consequently, *rapid, forced stretches are not recommended.*

Moving with less speed and more gently into a position does not cause such a reflex response. You will also find that as you hold a position the feeling of stretch actually subsides and you can move further into your stretch position. This is because a different reflex occurs. Specialized receptors in muscle tendons (called Golgi tendon organs) pick up information in the tendon about the amount of tension being applied by a muscle through its tendon. If there is a large amount of tension, as in a sustained *static* stretch, the reflex response is to *relax* the stretched muscle more fully — which means that you can move further into your stretch position. Static stretching techniques are also not associated with injury or damage to muscles or joints. Because of this, *static stretching techniques are recommended by many authorities for effectively increasing range of movement without causing injury.*

How long should you hold each stretch for? Here there is a difference of opinion, which seems to relate to your initial level of flexibility. If you are just beginning a stretching programme, holding each stretch for as little as ten seconds will cause marked improvements with regular stretching sessions (three or four per week) over a period of weeks. Yet it would appear that optimum stretch can be achieved with static stretches which are held for around thirty seconds each. If you are short of time, hold each stretch for the shorter period.

There are a number of variations of static stretching techniques, too. One very popular method is called *passive* stretching. In this technique it is common to employ gravity or the help of a partner to get you into a furthermost position. A gymnast doing the splits is an example of gravity aided passive stretching. A partner pressing on the inner thighs as in exercise 19 on page 43 causing the stretcher to go nearer to the floor, is a good example of partner-assisted passive stretching. Whilst passive stretching can be very effective, it also needs a lot of thought and control. It is relatively easy for a partner to become over zealous and cause injury, because he/she thinks you could go further! Your chosen partner must be sympathetic to your needs!

Another common stretching technique relies upon the fact that many researchers, though not all, have observed that muscles can relax more fully when they have been previously contracted. In this technique (which goes by the lengthy title of proprioceptive neuromuscular facilitation — or PNF for short) a muscle is contracted strongly before stretching — often you need the help of a partner for this. Then having held this contraction for a few seconds, you do your static stretch. Again the slight risk of injury is present because of the strong contraction against an object, yourself or partner, but this method has shown itself to be very effective.

Simplest of all the methods described though, is the static method of stretching and, arguably, it is also the most effective especially if each stretch is *eased into, held, and further eased into if the stretch subsides, for a total of thirty seconds.* Whilst you are stretching do ensure that the rest of your body is as relaxed possible.

Summary of stretching guidelines

All stretches should be anatomically possible.

All stretches need to suit you.

For the best stretch, warm up first.

Use preparatory stretching towards the end of your warm-up (if going on to further exercise).

All stretches should feel comfortable.

All stretches should be progressive.

Avoid forced or bounced movements.

Ease into a stretch, then hold each stretch for a minimum of ten seconds, but preferably for thirty seconds.

Following more strenuous exercise your body is very warm — do the bulk of your stretching now.

Use partner stretching intelligently and sympathetically.

Assessing yourself _____

Most people can begin a stretch programme like the ones outlined in this book
without any problem. However, as with any exercise programme, it is wise to ask yourself a few
questions first. If you can answer 'yes' to any of the following questions, you are advised to get specialist advice,
including medical clearance from your GP before you begin:

1. Has your doctor ever told you that you have high blood pressure, or any cardiovascular problem?

2. Is there any history of heart disease in your family?

3. Have you ever been troubled by unaccountable chest pain, or tightness in the chest, especially if associated with minimal effort?

4. Are you prone to headaches, fainting or dizziness?

5. Have you any medical condition which you think might interfere with your participation in an exercise programme?

6. Do you suffer from pain or limited movement in any joint?

7. Are you taking any drugs or medication at the moment?

8. Are you extremely overweight, or extremely underweight?

9. Are you a newcomer to exercise and over 40?

10. Are you pregnant?

How flexible are you?
One very simple test of your general flexibility is known as the sit and reach test. Essentially the test assesses your lower back and hamstring flexibility, but this would seem to be a good indicator of your general range of movement.

Equipment needed for the test:
1 cardboard box
1 ruler
sticky tape.

This is a do-it-yourself version of what is normally used, but it is just as accurate as the ready-made reaching box, and much cheaper!

All that you need to do is tape the ruler to the middle of your cardboard box as illustrated:

Now place the box against a wall.

Position yourself with your feet flat against the box as in the diagram

Keeping your legs straight, knees flat on the floor, reach forward with outstretched arms — do not jerk forward! *Ease* as far forward as you can, noting where you are in relationship to the ruler and your toes. Are you close to your feet — if so, how close? Have you gone past your toes — if so by how much?

Make a note of the number of inches or centimetres in front of, or past your toes that your fingertips are. Record this measurement. It will serve as a guide to how effective your stretching programme is, when you re-test yourself at a subsequent date (say in three months' time).

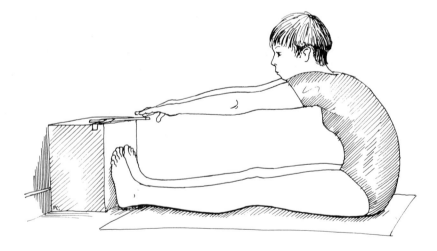

Your stretching programme _____

Warm up

The importance of warming up thoroughly has already been stressed in the stretching guidelines on page 10, where the methods of warming up have also been described.

The sequence of exercises in this section has been designed to generally mobilize the major joints of the body and warm the large muscle groups. It should be followed by anyone who intends to carry out a comprehensive stretching routine.

The exercises can also be used in other ways. If you are a keen jogger or runner, the sequence will also serve as a general joint mobilizing session, which coupled with some preparatory stretches (see PROGRAMMES on page 58) will fully prepare your body for your running session. The bulk of your stretching can then be carried out after your run. The same goes for other sports too. Refer to PROGRAMMES to see what is recommended for other activities.

Likewise, if you intend to do just a few stretches for a specific part of the body, you may only need to do a few specific exercises from the mobilizing section. Once again, refer to PROGRAMMES for guidance.

1

Mobilizers

Posture

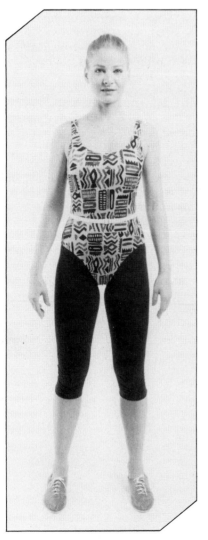

Start by checking your posture. Your feet should be a comfortable distance apart, about hip width, with weight evenly balanced. Some people find it more comfortable to have the feet pointing out slightly.

Your pelvis should feel 'centred' — with your bottom not sticking out, but tucked under slightly.

Spine should be long, shoulders down away from your ears.

Have your arms loosely by your sides and look forward.

Feel tall, but not rigid.

Breathe comfortably and start thinking about your exercise and stretching programme.

2 & 3

Shoulder circles
(alternate and double)

Standing with good posture and keeping your arms down, raise your right shoulder up towards your ear, take it back and then down again in a circular movement. Repeat the movement, keeping a steady rhythm, 12 times, then change sides, repeating the sequence with the left shoulder.

Breathe comfortably throughout.

Now perform the exercise as before, this time circling both shoulders at once.
Repeat 12 times.

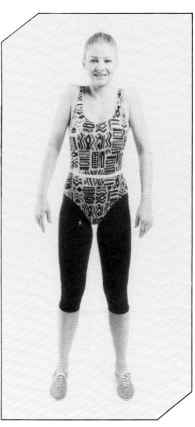

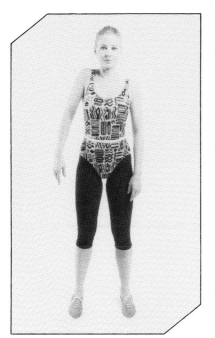

4 & 5

Arm circles
(alternate and double)

Stand tall with good posture. Raise one arm forward, take it up and back, still keeping a good distance between your shoulder and your ear.

Keep your spine long throughout. Repeat 12 times on each side, breathing comfortably throughout.

Repeat the exercise as before, using both arms together.

Avoid the tendency to arch the spine.

Repeat 12 times.

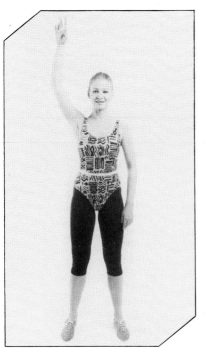 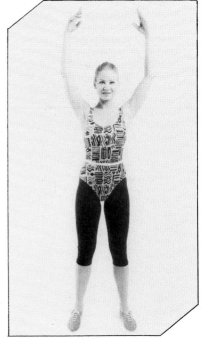

6

Side bends

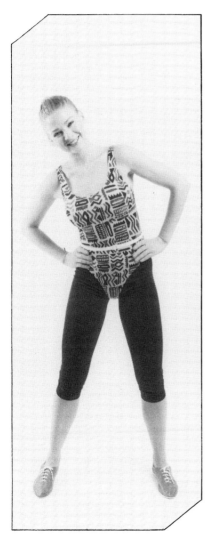

Stand tall with good posture. Place hands on hips and take feet slightly wider apart to give you a more stable base.

Keeping your spine long, lift up and away from your hips, before bending over to first one side, then the other. Do not lean forwards or backwards.

Repeat 12 times on each side, breathing out as you bend to the side, and in as you return.

7

Waist twists

Stand tall with good posture.
Take your feet slightly wider apart and bend your knees just a little. Bring your arms up in front of you, bent at the elbow.

Keeping your spine long, try and turn your shoulders round to the side, while still keeping your hips facing forwards.

Keep the movement smooth, breathing easily throughout the sequence.

Repeat 12 times on each side.

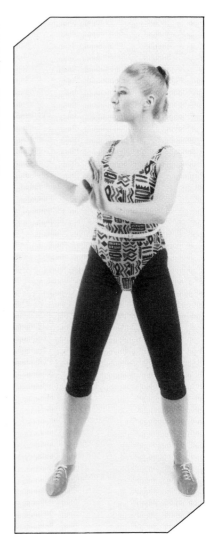

8

Rib isolations

Stand tall with good posture, then raise your arms out to the side at shoulder level.

Keep your spine long and your hips stable and facing forwards.

Now take your ribcage first to the left then to the right.

Breathe comfortably throughout, repeating each movement 12 times on each side.

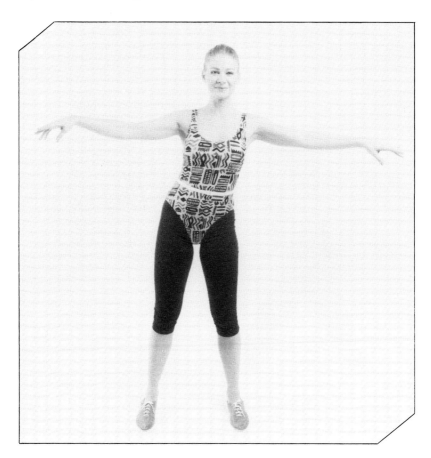

9

Ceiling reaches

Stand tall with good posture. Take your feet slightly wider apart. Keep your spine long and reach up for the ceiling with your left arm, bending your left knee at the same time so that you feel a stretch down the left side of the trunk. (Make sure that your knee follows the same line as your foot).

Repeat 12 times on each side, alternating the exercise with a flowing rhythm.

Breathe comfortably throughout.

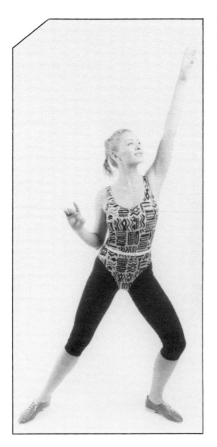

10

Pliés

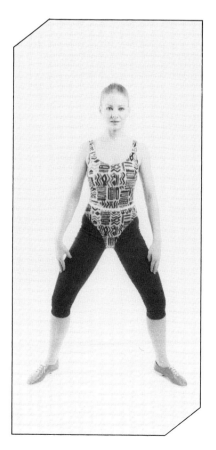

Stand tall with good posture
Take the feet a little wider, and
turn the legs out from the hips.
Now bend the knees, keeping
them following the same line as
your feet. Keep your spine long and
your bottom tucked under.

Go down as far as you can without lifting your heels off the ground,
then fully straighten and repeat 24
times, breathing easily throughout.

11

Skiing

Stand tall with good posture. Reach up with both arms until they are high above your head, then swing them smoothly down by your sides, bending your knees at the same time.

Keep your back long and your knees following the same line as your toes. Continue going down towards the floor until your hands brush the ground, then swing back up to your starting position.

Breathe in as you descend, and out as you rise, repeating the whole sequence 24 times.

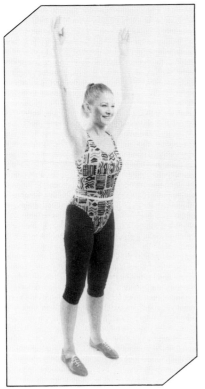 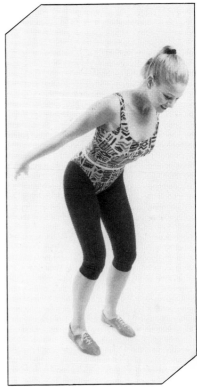

Having completed some general mobilizing, move on to some large muscle group activity to get really warm. Jogging in place is outlined here, but remember there are lots of options: indoor cycling, re-bounding, treadmill running, etc.

Remember not to make this activity too intense or too long. As part of a warm up phase, 3 to 5 minutes of light activity is enough. You should only be slightly out of breath and just starting to glow!

If you are really blowing hard, your exercise was too intense, and you should keep moving your limbs at a much reduced pace until you are feeling less stressed. Remember that it is dangerous to stop still following strenuous exercise—keep moving slowly and rhythmically using the same muscles that you were using in the exercise but at a much lower intensity. For instance, if you have been running, bring your activity down to a walk, until you are breathing almost normally.

12

Jogging

If you are limited for space, you can still jog in place. Keep your spine long, let your arms swing loosely by your sides and use the whole of your foot in the jogging action. Begin by 'padding' through the floor, peeling one foot off the floor at a time. Increase the range of movement gradually, still making sure that you always put your heel down on the floor with each step.

If you intend to jog for any length of time, the correct shoes will prevent excessive pounding of your feet.

For a light warm up, as part of this sequence, 3 to 5 minutes of light padding or low jogging is ample.

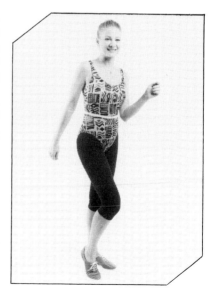

Your stretching programmes

The stretches

Read each set of instructions for the stretches you are going to do very carefully. It is important that you position yourself correctly if you are going to get an efficient 'safe stretch'.

Unless you are doing preparatory stretches, or are very pressed for time, hold each stretch position for approximately thirty seconds. Do move further into your stretch position if the feeling of stretch subsides while you are maintaining your position. Working like this will give you the best results.

If you are aiming to get rapid results from your stretch programme, make sure that you follow all the guidelines given earlier (summary on page 14) and try and stretch regularly at least every other day.

If you are stretching as part of your fitness or training programme, include preparatory stretches before your fitness or training session (where appropriate), but do the bulk of your stretching work at the end of your activity session.

The instructions are quite precise and nearly always begin with the words 'Stand or sit tall with good posture'. This is because to get the most from each stretch you need to be in the right starting position — and that means good posture. Standing tall means just that — and you should refer back to the posture pointers on page 18 of the mobilizing section. Sitting tall means that you should aim for a long spine with your shoulders back and down, head balanced with neck long. Really feel as if you are perched high on your 'sitting bones' with your pelvis centred and tummy in.

Where specific instructions are given for getting into a stretch position, repeat the instructions in reverse order for getting out of that position.

Remember that with each stretch you should go as far into the stretch as you can, without compromising any of the technical guidelines. Once into the stretch, hold that furthermost position. Listen to your body at all times.

For most of the stretches you should breathe normally unless you are otherwise instructed. Avoid the tendency to hold your breath throughout the whole of the exercise. Some people find that it is easier to move further into a stretch if you breath out at the same time. Try it, and if it works for you, do it.

Concentrating on what you are doing helps tremendously. Really think about the body parts you are stretching as you do each exercise. This technique is known as visualization and is used with great success by many world class sportsmen and women.

Whilst you are stretching, do try and keep the rest of your body relaxed, so as not to build up unnecessary tension in other muscle groups.

Having stretched, some people like to shake out the stretched limbs loosely. If this works for you, do it.

Do dress warmly — loose layers of clothing are ideal. Make sure that you can move easily and freely in whatever you are wearing.

If you are going to wear shoes, they should be very pliable. Most stretches do not need footwear, unless you are exercising on a rough or splintered floor. In this event lay down a mat or large bath towel to protect yourself during the floor, seated or floor-lying exercises. Exercising on carpet can produce carpet 'burns', so a mat or towel might be advisable in this case as well.

1

Head turns

Stand or sit tall with good posture. Keep your spine long and your shoulders away from your ears as you turn your head as far to the right as it will go. Hold this position, keeping your chin parallel to your shoulder — you will feel the stretch in the side of your neck.

Repeat on the other side.

Breathe easily throughout.

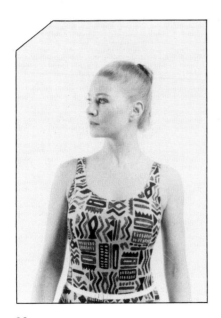

Head tilts 1 & 2

1 Stand or sit tall with good posture, keeping your spine long and your shoulders down away from your ears. Maintaining a long neck, tilt your head to the side as far as it will go — you will feel the stretch in the side of your neck and the top of your opposite shoulder.

Repeat on the other side.
Breathe easily throughout.

2 The head tilts exercise can be made more difficult by placing the left hand on top of the head when tilting to the left and by placing the right hand on top of the head when tilting to the right.

The hand provides extra weight which increases the stretch. It should be loosely rested on top of the head and not used to pull the head down.

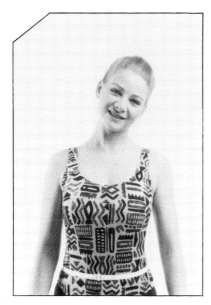
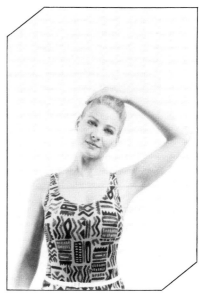

4 & 5

Head forward 1 & 2

1   Stand or sit tall with good posture, keeping your spine long, shoulders down and tummy tucked in. Maintaining a long neck, bring your chin towards your chest, feeling the stretch along the back of your neck. Hold your furthermost position.

Breathe easily throughout.

2   As with the head tilt exercise, increase the head forward stretch by adding extra weight in the form of your hands loosely resting on top your head. Do not pull!

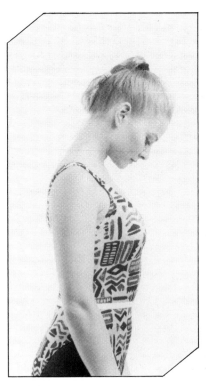 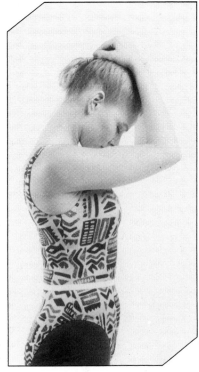

6

Diagonal stretch

Stand or sit tall with good posture. Keep your spine long and your shoulders down away from your ears. Maintaining a long neck, turn your head to look along a diagonal, then tilt your head by bringing your chin towards your chest, feeling the stretch in the back of the neck and upper back.

Breathe easily throughout.

Increase the stretch by resting your hand loosely on the top of your head.

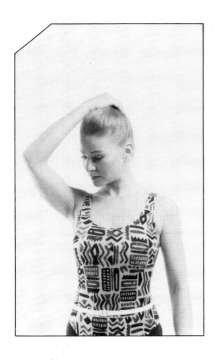

7

Upper back stretch

Stand tall with good posture. Bend your knees slightly and tilt your pelvis under.

Now interlock your fingers, pushing your hands away from your chest, and round off your upper back, tilting your head to look down at the same time.

You will feel the stretch between your shoulder blades, and in your lower back.

Breathe easily throughout.

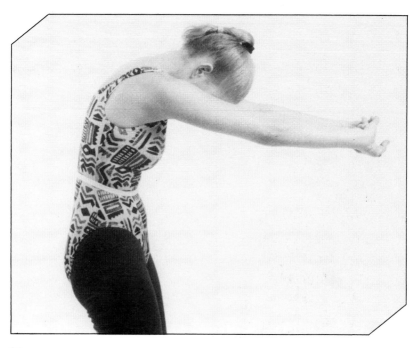

8

Shoulder stretch

Stand tall with good posture. Keeping your spine long and your shoulders down away from your ears, take one arm up and behind you, and the other one down and behind you.

Aim to clasp your fingers together. You will feel the stretch around the shoulders, side and chest.

Repeat on both sides, breathing easily throughout.

If this exercise is difficult because you are unable to clasp your fingers, hold a belt or towel in the upper hand, then reach behind to grasp the belt with your other hand, then gradually inch your hands closer together.

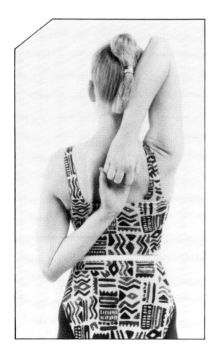

9

Shoulder and side stretch

Stand tall with good posture. Keep your spine long and your shoulders away from your ears. Now raise both arms up and use the hand of the right arm, placed behind the elbow of the left arm, to bring the left upper arm behind your head.

You will feel the stretch in the shoulder and side of the trunk.

Repeat on both sides, breathing easily throughout.

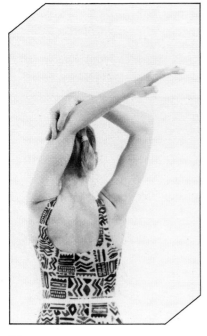

10 & 11

Chest stretch 1 & 2

1 Stand tall with good posture side on to a wall, with one foot forward for balance.

Keeping your shoulders down and spine long, place an outstretched arm flat against the wall at shoulder height. (You may have to turn to face the wall to do this.)

Now try to turn so that your shoulders are facing forwards.

You will feel the stretch in the chest and front of shoulder.

Repeat on both sides, breathing easily throughout.

2 Stand tall with good posture. Place your hands loosely clasped on the small of your back.

Keeping your spine long and your shoulders down, try and bring your elbows together. You will feel the stretch in the chest.

Breathe easily throughout.

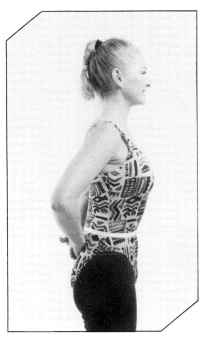

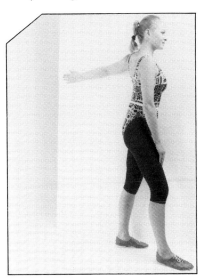

12

Side stretch 1

1 Stand tall with good posture. Now take your feet slightly wider apart to give a more stable base and rest both hands on your hips.

Keeping your spine long and your shoulders down away from your ears, lift up from your hips and bend to the side as far as possible.

You will feel the stretch down the side of your waist.

Repeat on the other side.

Breathe comfortably throughout.

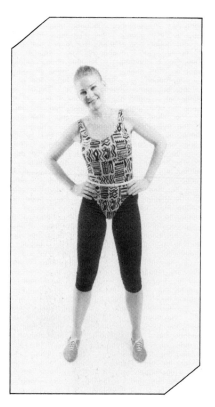

13 & 14

Side stretch 2 & 3

2 The side stretch can be made progressively harder by taking one arm above your head.

3 The side stretch is harder still with both arms raised.

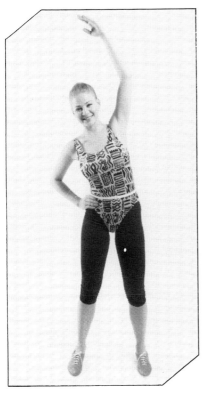 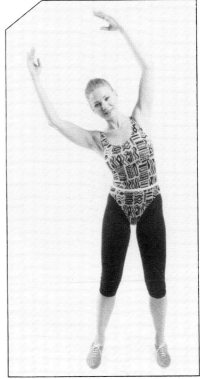

15

Spine and trunk twist

Sit upright on the floor with your legs out in front of you.

Bend the right leg up in front of you, placing the right foot on the outside of the left knee.

Keeping the spine long and the shoulders away from the ears, twist round so that your shoulders face forward.

You may find it useful to lever yourself slightly using your left elbow against your right knee.

Use your right arm for balance.

You will feel the stretch right through the trunk and spine.

Repeat on both sides, breathing easily throughout.

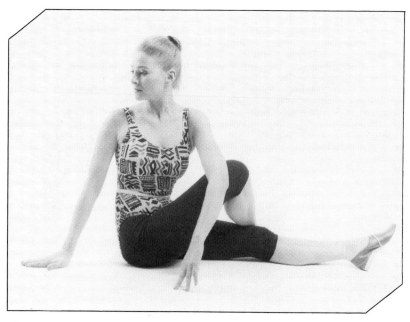

16

Seated groin stretch 1

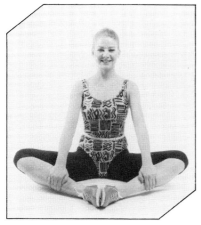

1   Sit tall with good posture. Bend your legs up towards you with soles of your feet together and allow your knees to fall out towards the floor.

Keep your spine long and your shoulders away from your ears.

Rest your hands on your calves, or ankles. If you find it difficult to sit upright in this position, use your hands behind you for balance.

You will feel the stretch along the insides of your thighs and groin.

Breathe easily throughout.

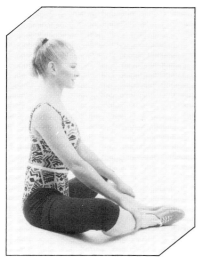

Seated groin stretch 2 & 3

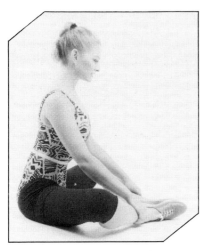

2 To increase the stretch and to stretch the hamstrings at the same time, keep a long spine and hinge forward from your hips as far as you can, holding your furthermost position.

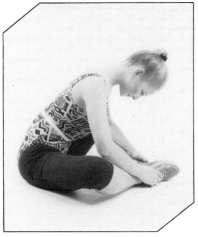

3 From your hinged position relax your back. You will then find that you can move further forward. Go as far forward as possible feeling more stretch in the backs of the buttocks and thighs. Hold your furthermost position.

19

Lying groin stretch

Lie flat on the floor, pressing your lower back firmly into the ground as you slide both legs up towards you. Place the soles of your feet together and allow your knees to fall out loosely to the floor.

You will feel the stretch in the inner thigh and groin.

Breathe easily throughout.

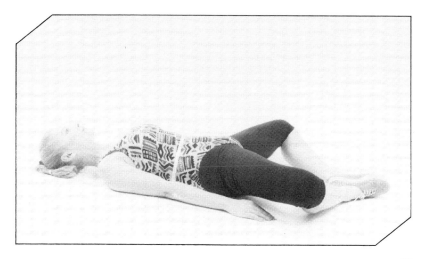

20

Dancers' stretch 1

1 Sit tall with good posture with legs outstretched. Gradually take your legs out to the side in a large 'V', but still keeping legs straight. Only take your legs out as far as is comfortable and use your hands behind you to help you keep your back upright.

You will feel the stretch along the inner thigh and groin.

Breathe easily throughout.

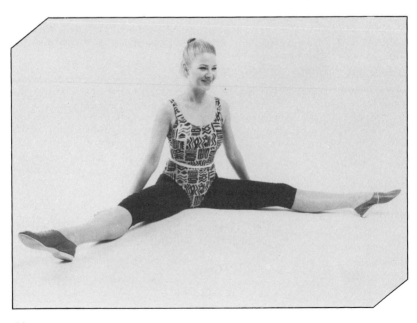

21 & 22

Dancers'
stretch 2 & 3

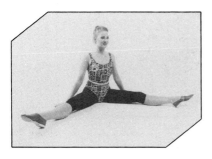

2   Now try and hinge forward from the position achieved in stretch 19, keeping your back straight. Go as far as you can and hold your furthermost position.

(In both these stretches vary the position of your feet from flexed to pointed, noting the different sensations of stretch.)

3   From the position achieved in stretch 20 it is possible to carry out many other variations which affect the backs of the legs, buttocks and spine differently.

Reaching towards the left foot, right foot and centre for example, with flexed or pointed feet and rounded or straight back. Use these to add variety.

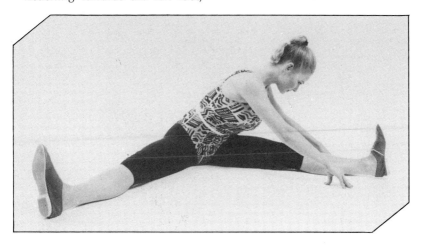

23

Lying hamstring stretch

Lie flat on the floor. Slide both feet along the floor until both knees are at an angle of 90°. Keep your back flat against the floor, especially the lower back.

Now raise the left leg, grasping it loosely behind the thigh with both hands. Straighten your leg fully, then bring your leg as close to your chest as possible, still keeping it straight and keeping your shoulders down, your neck long, and lower back flat. You will feel the stretch along the back of the leg.

Experiment with a flexed and a pointed foot, noting the difference in sensation.

Repeat on both sides, breathing easily throughout.

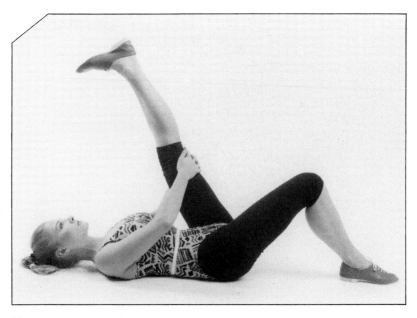

24

Standing hamstring stretch

Stand tall with good posture. Bend at the knees and hips until you can easily rest your chest on your thighs. Reach round with your arms and grasp your calves to bring your chest and thighs firmly together.

From this position, try to straighten your legs smoothly, whilst still keeping your chest firmly against the thighs.

You will feel the stretch along the back of the legs.

Breathe easily throughout.

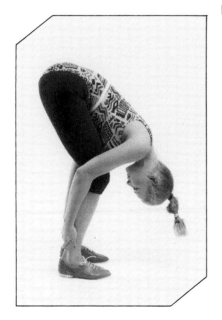

25

Lying quadriceps stretch

Lie face down on the floor, resting your forehead on your right hand.

Press your hips firmly into the floor and bend your left foot up towards your buttocks.

Reach round with your left arm to gently ease your left foot closer to your buttocks. You will feel the stretch in the front of the left thigh.

Repeat on both sides, breathing easily throughout.

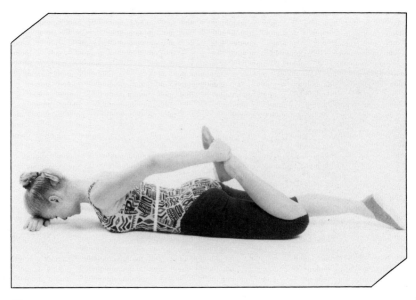

26

Standing quadriceps stretch

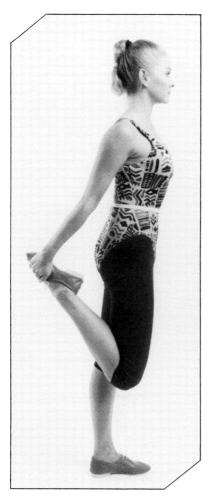

Stand tall with good posture. Holding a chair back for support, reach behind you with your right arm to loosely grasp your right foot.

Smoothly ease your foot towards your buttocks whilst keeping your spine long and your bottom tucked under.

Keep your shoulders down and neck long. You will feel the stretch in the front of the right thigh.

Repeat on both sides, breathing easily throughout.

27 & 28

Standing calf stretch 1 & 2

1 Stand tall with one leg in front of the other supporting your weight and resting your palms at shoulder height on a wall or firm support.

From this position, ease your back leg out behind you, keeping it fully straight, heel pressed into the floor, hips parallel and facing forward. Keep your spine as long as possible with shoulders down. You should feel the stretch in the calf of your back leg. If not, ease your leg further behind you, still making sure that your heel is pressed firmly into the floor.

Repeat on both sides, breathing easily throughout.

2 To stretch the calf lower down, adopt the same position as before, but bend your back leg slightly, keeping the heel pressed into the floor and hold.

Repeat on both sides breathing easily throughout.

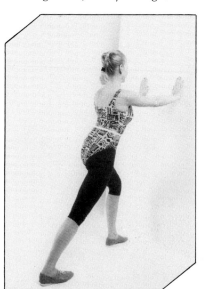 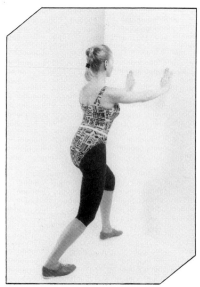

29

Lying hip and thigh stretch

Lie flat on your back with your lower back pressed into the floor. Bring your right knee up to your chest, holding it there with loosely clasped hands. Keep your other leg firmly stretched out along the floor with foot flexed. You will feel the stretch along the front of the thigh and around the hip and buttocks.

Repeat on both sides, breathing easily throughout.

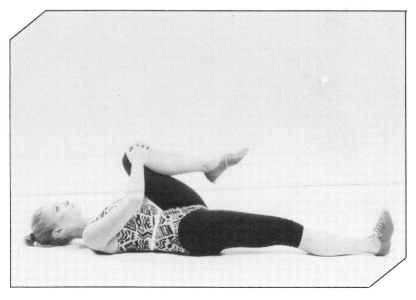

30

Standing hip and thigh stretch

Stand tall with good posture in front of a firm chair or stool. Raise one foot up on to the chair back, easing your body slowly towards this foot so that chest and thigh come closer together. Rest your hands loosely on the raised knee and keep your spine and back leg straight and shoulders down.

Ease as far forward as possible, then hold. You will feel the stretch along the front of the thigh and around the hip and buttocks.

Repeat on both sides, breathing easily throughout.

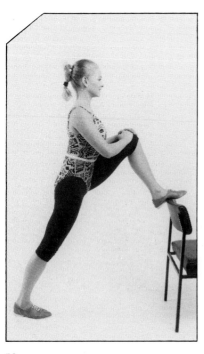

31

Back release

Lie flat on your back, then slide your knees up to your chest, hugging them close to your chest with loosely clasped hands. Feel the stretch in the lower back. Breathe easily throughout.

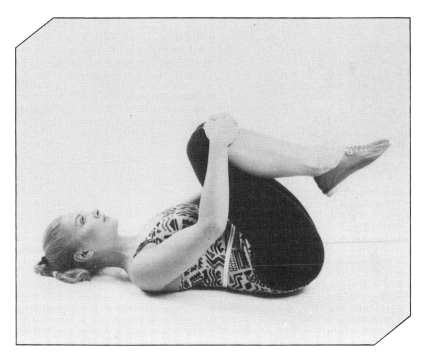

Seated hamstring stretch 1 & 2

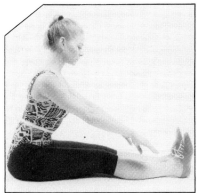

1 Sit tall on the floor with legs outstretched. (If it is not possible to sit up straight with legs straight, bend your knees until your back is straight.)

Keeping your spine long and shoulders down, hinge forward at your hips and reach towards your flexed feet.

You will feel the stretch in the backs of your legs and you will also feel the muscles in your back working strongly to maintain your upright position.

If you are having problems reaching forward, a belt or towel looped around the feet can help you achieve a greater stretch.

Breathe easily throughout.

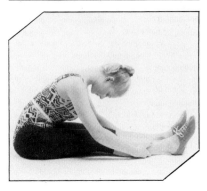

2 Sit tall on the floor, legs outstretched as in the previous exercise.

Follow the guidelines given for the earlier hamstring stretch, but this time allow your back to relax, so that your chest comes nearer to your thighs.

You will feel the stretch in the backs of the legs.

Breathe easily throughout.

34 & 35

Seated hamstring and groin stretch 1 & 2

1 Sit tall with both legs fully outstretched. Bend your right leg so that your right foot rests along your inner thigh, with your right knee as close to the floor as possible.

Keeping your spine long and your shoulders away from your ears, hinge forwards from the hips reaching for your flexed left foot.

You will feel the stretch in the back of your left leg and in the groin. You will also feel your back muscles working strongly to maintain your upright spine.

As with previous seated exercises, use a belt or towel looped around your foot to help you inch further forward.

Repeat on both sides, breathing easily throughout.

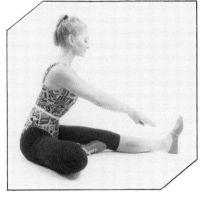

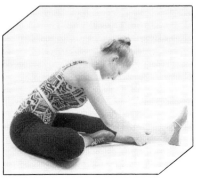

2 The previous exercise can be varied by rounding the back and bringing the chest nearer the thigh. Again, breathe easily throughout.

Back and hamstring stretch/strengthener 1 & 2

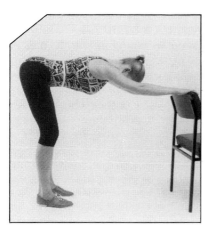

1 Stand tall with good posture a comfortable distance away from the back of a chair or table top.

Bend at the knees and hips and reach forwards with your arms to grasp the chair back (or table top).

Now try and straighten your back as much as possible so that you have a straight line from tail to head.

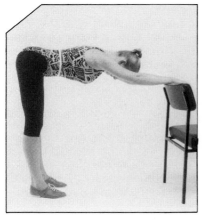

2 If you can, gradually straighten your legs from the position achieved in the previous exercise still keeping your back flat.

You will feel the stretch in the backs of your legs and a lot of muscular work going on trying to keep your back flat.

Breathe easily throughout.

38

Front of trunk stretch

Lie fully outstretched, face down on the floor.

Bring your arms to your sides to give support and gradually ease you chest off the floor, whilst still keeping your hips firmly pressed into the floor.

You will feel the stretch in the front of the trunk.

Breathe easily throughout.

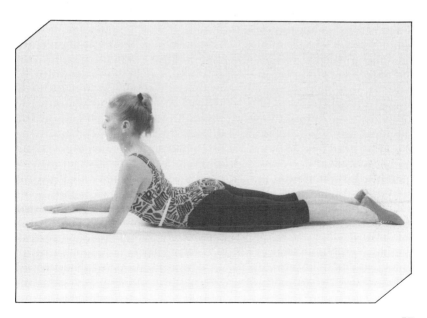

Sample programmes___

This section gives suggested programmes for various activities and sports. If you find that other exercises not listed in your programme suit your purposes better, then by all means include them in your routine.

Comprehensive stretching programme

There are many variations of a general overall stretching programme which could be given using the exercises included in this book. The following programme is a suggestion only. Modify the programme according to your needs, obviously trying to ensure that all areas of the body are included. Always make sure that you mobilize and warm up thoroughly first.

Complete mobilizers **1-11**.

Carry out a few minutes of large muscle group activity at low intensity, like jogging.

Perform the following stretches (numbers refer to listing in the previous chapter):

1	Head turn	**16**	Seated groin stretch 1
2	Head tilt 1	**23**	Lying hamstring stretch
4	Head forward 1	**25**	Lying quadriceps stretch
6	Diagonal stretch	**29**	Hip and back stretch
7	Upper back stretch	**31**	Back release
9	Shoulder and side stretch	**33**	Seated hamstring stretch
11	Chest stretch	**38**	Front and trunk stretch
12	Side stretch 1	**27**	Calf stretch 1
15	Spine and trunk twist	**28**	Calf stretch 2

Hold each stretch for thirty seconds.

Repeat the whole sequence regularly every other day.

The programme can be made more demanding if required by adding more stretches as appropriate. Some people like to hold the stretches for longer as they progress, but no great further changes seem to occur when compared against the thirty second stretches.

Remember your stretching programme will always be progressive if you attempt to move as far as possible into the stretch and hold it without sacrificing technique.

Runner's stretch
Whilst it is true that most runners can just get up and run, mobilizing first can be very beneficial, especially if a few preparatory stretches are included. Move smoothly from one stretch to the next.

Complete mobilizers **1-11**

Perform preparatory stretches:

24	Standing hamstring stretch	**16**	Seated groin stretch
26	Standing quadriceps stretch	**23**	Lying hamstring stretch
30	Hip and thigh stretch	**35**	Seated hamstring and groin stretch
27	Calf stretch 1	**38**	Front trunk stretch
28	Calf stretch 2	**31**	Back release

(Hold preparatory stretches for ten seconds)

On your return from your run, allow your body to return nearer normal, but keep moving, then carry out a general stretch such as suggested on page 58 (Comprehensive stretching programme).

Cyclist's stretch
Complete mobilizers **1-11**, moving smoothly from one to the next.

Perform preparatory stretches:

1	Head turn	**24**	Standing hamstring stretch
4	Head forward	**26**	Standing quadriceps stretch
9	Shoulder and side stretch	**30**	Hip and thigh stretch
11	Chest stretch	**36**	Back and hamstring stretch
12	Side stretch	**27**	Calf stretch 1
15	Spine and trunk twist	**28**	Calf stretch 2

(Hold preparatory stretches for ten seconds each)

On your return from your ride, carry out a general stretch as suggested on page 58.

Swimmer's stretch

Complete mobilizers **1-11**, moving smoothly from one to the next.

Perform preparatory stretches:

7	Upper back stretch	**17**	Seated groin stretch
8	Shoulder stretch	**23**	Lying hamstring stretch
9	Shoulder and side stretch	**25**	Lying quadriceps stretch
10	Chest stretch	**29**	Hip and back stretch
12	Side stretch	**31**	Back release
15	Spine and trunk twist	**38**	Front and trunk stretch

(Hold preparatory stretches for ten seconds each)

After your swim, keep warm and carry out a general stretch programme as suggested on page 58.

Weight trainer's stretch

Weight training can be made more efficient and safer with an appropriate warm up including preparatory stretching.

Complete mobilizers **1-11**

Perform preparatory stretches:

7	Upper back stretch	**29**	Hip and back stretch
9	Shoulder and side stretch	**32**	Seated hamstring stretch
11	Chest stretch	**38**	Front of trunk stretch
12	Side stretch	**31**	Back release
15	Spine and trunk twist	**26**	Standing quadriceps stretch
16	Seated groin stretch	**27**	Calf stretch 1
23	Lying hamstring stretch	**28**	Calf stretch 2

(Hold preparatory stretches for ten seconds)

Then go on to large muscle group exercises of low intensity.

After your weight training session, carry out a general stretch such as suggested on page 58.

If you train on a split routine of any sort, modify your stretching accordingly, stretching only those body parts which you will be working.

Sample programmes ___
Posture

Two of the most common faulty postures are illustrated below.

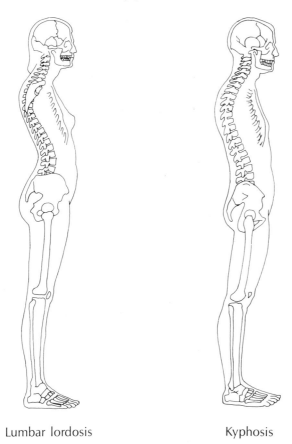

Lumbar lordosis   Kyphosis

Both postures often cause other ailments and are associated with pain in more extreme cases. Both can also be helped through stretching.

Lordosis programme
Complete mobilizers **1-11**.

Perform stretches:

31 Back release

33 Seated hamstring stretch
(back release)

23 Lying hamstring stretch

29 Lying hip and back stretcher

36 Back and hamstring stretch
strengthener

Hold each position for thirty seconds, repeating the whole sequence three times. Repeat the programme every other day. When this feels comfortable move on to a general programme.

Certain strengthening exercises can also help this condition. For a detailed explanation of such exercises and how to implement them into your programme, see *Shape your body, shape your life,* published by Patrick Stephens Ltd, price £3.99.

Kyphosis programme
Complete mobilizers **1-11**.

Perform stretches:

10 Chest stretch 1

11 Chest stretch 2

Because kyphosis tends to be associated with lordosis, complete the exercises from this programme, too.

Hold each position for thirty seconds, repeating the whole sequence three times. When this feels comfortable, move on to a general programme.

As with lordosis, certain strengthening exercises may help. Again for detailed information, see *Shape your body, shape your life.*

Typist's stretch
This short programme is for anyone who finds themselves seated for long periods of time in front of a typewriter, VDU or desk.

It can be carried out in the office.

Complete mobilizers **2-5**

Perform stretches:

7 Upper back stretch

8 Shoulder stretch

9 Shoulder and side stretch

10 Chest stretch 1

11 Chest stretch 2

1 Head turn

6 Diagonal stretch

You may also find any of the neck exercises useful (**1-6** inclusive).

Hold each stretch for thirty seconds. Repeat the sequence whenever you feel that you have been sitting still for too long in the same position.

Supplement with a general programme carried out regularly.

Cramp
Cramp can often be relieved by stretching out the muscles which are going into spasm. The calf is a common site for cramp attacks. Use exercises **27** and **28** immediately!

Other areas can also be dealt with by the appropriate stretch.

Muscle soreness

Delayed onset muscle soreness is common after unaccustomed or over-strenuous physical activity. Stretching can relieve the problem to a certain extent, but you must warm up thoroughly.

If the problem is general, complete the mobilizers plus a warming routine like jogging slowly for a few minutes. Then carry out a general stretch programme. If the soreness is more specific, warm up thoroughly, then chose the appropriate exercises.

Headache programme

Some people find that stretching helps relieve tension headaches. Here is a typical stretching programme for such sufferers.

Complete mobilizers **2-5**.

Perform exercises:

1 Head turn
2 Head tilt 1
3 Head tilt 2
4 Head forward 2

5 Head forward 2
6 Diagonal stretch
7 Upper back stretch

Hold each stretch for thirty seconds. Repeat the sequence as appropriate.

Supplement with a general programme carried out regularly.

Period pain

Depending upon the type and nature of your period pain, certain exercises seem to help.

Complete mobilizers **1-11**.

Perform stretches:

31 Back release

30 Hip and thigh stretch (standing)

29 Hip and back stretch (lying)

19 Lying groin stretch

Hold each stretch for thirty seconds. Repeat as appropriate.